ALL YOU NEED TO KNOW ABOUT CERVICAL CANCER

JACKSON BOOM

COMPREHENSIVE KNOWLEDGE ABOUT CERVICAL CANCER...

Abstract

Cancer as all of us realize is a malignant increase or replication of cells abnormally in an organ or tissue. Cancer is among the sector's deadliest illnesses that kill hundreds of human beings throughout the globe. The threat of survival is narrow particularly if now no longer detected early.

Cancers start with modifications in a cellular or organization of cells; those adjustments have an effect on the ordinary cells thereby   main to their out of control replication ensuing to lump or tumor formation (malignant tumor). Malignancy of a tumor way that they are able to unfold to close by tissues and preserve growing. NOTE that a few most cancers cells can break up, input the blood and are carried to a far off tissue wherein it begins to evolve to develop and shape new tumors. While now no longer in itself a sexually transmitted disorder, cervical most cancers is connected to the presence of the human papilloma virus, that's sexually transmitted. Survival quotes are notably better wherein analysis is early, and a countrywide screening programme has decreased mortality withinside the UK. However, uptake is low in a few companies and nurses have a function in growing uptake. The NHS cervical screening programme gives screening to all ladies elderly 25 to sixty five and monitors 3.7 million girls every year (Department of Health, 2003). About seven percent of those have a few abnormality requiring follow-up (Wright et al, 2002). In many instances ladies can be reassured that the abnormality is not going to development and that no remedy - other than near surveillance - is required. A small wide variety may be informed that their hassle is extra serious, and a percentage of those could be identified with cervical most cancers. Cervical most cancers is the 1/3 most deadly cancers in girls, with a demise price of 231,000 a yr worldwide. It killed 1,123 ladies withinside the UK in 2002 - approximately 3.7 in step with 100,000. However, the loss of life charge in growing international locations is extensively better at 5-15 in line with 100,000 (O'Meara, 2002). This article discusses the levels of cervical abnormality and examines the function of human papilloma virus (HPV) and cervical intraepithelial neoplasia (CIN). It additionally examines control of cell abnormalities and most cancers remedy and nurses' function in elevating uptake of screening.

Presentation and danger elements (risk factors)

The cervix is the distal(inferior) a part of the uterus, which protrudes into the vagina. It is made and based through styles of epithelium: {1}the endocervical epithelium which strains the uterus and advanced a part of the cervix, and {2} the squamous epithelium that is positioned distal to the endocervical epithelium. The epithelia cells terminates in a area referred to as the transformation zone, in which maximum cell abnormalities arise. Cervical most cancers can increase from the squamous cells or endocervical epithelium, however squamous cellular carcinomas are the most common and account for 85-ninety in line with cent of the sector cervical malignancies The common age of presentation is fifty four years, even though intraepithelial lesions are frequently recognized at a miles in advance age suggesting lengthy latency among mobile abnormality and malignancy The most common symptom of cervical most cancers is extraordinary bleeding occasionally among periods, after intercourse .This can be followed through offensive vaginal discharge.

Risk elements consist of:

-Smoking cigarettes

-Infection with HPV

-Use of contraceptives over a protracted duration of time

-Exposure to a few pills in the course of being pregnant like diethylstilbestrol

- Multiple sexual partners (or a sexual courting with a person who has had a couple of partners);

- Smoking;

- Immuno suppression.

Women that present the symptom early earlier than the most cancers will become too superior have the quality diagnosis and prognosis; cervical screening is powerful due to the fact cervical most cancers has an extended pre-invasive segment.

Symptom of cervical cancers

The signs/symptoms can be related to different medical conditions. But it's far recommended to look your physician when you have or enjoy any of the subsequent signs and symptoms;

- Vaginal bleeding even after intercourse
- Pelvic ache
- Pain in the course of sexual intercourse
- Abnormal vaginal discharges

Cervical most cancers screening

Cervical most cancers screening differs from breast screening, which makes use of mammography to hit upon most cancers in its early levels. Cervical cytology targets to stumble on precancerous cells or tissues [lesions] and deal with them earlier than they turn out to be malignant. The NHS Cervical Screening Programme became released withinside the Nineteen Nineties for the motive of slicing down the price of mortality from cervical most cancers by 20 percent or extra.

Cervical smears

In order to discover cellular adjustments a cervical smear ('Pap' smear) is completed. Until currently this changed into the mainstay of the screening programme, even though new technology have because been introduced. The cervical smear includes gathering cells from the suspected hotspot zone, typically the use of a aggregate of endocervical brush and spatula. Samples are gathered and placed [smeared] directly to a slide, constant with a cytology fixative after which despatched for laboratory evaluation through cytologists. While easy and comparatively inexpensive, the cervical smear isn't perfect. False bad consequences are yielded as a minimum 20 in keeping with cent of the time- -thirds of which might be resulting from sampling or education mistakes. There is likewise a 5 consistent with cent fake effective fee. It's fake poor or high-quality end result can be related to mistakes in training or contaminations with ordinary cells.

Liquid-primarily based cytology

Because of the shortcomings of the smear check, this led the National Institute for Clinical Excellence to suggest using liquid-primarily based totally cytology (LBC), wherein the pattern is amassed in a comparable manner, however the head of the spatula is snapped off and rinsed in preservative fluid. This is transported to a laboratory in which it's far processed to do away with unneeded cloth and the consequent cell suspension is transferred to a slide and stained. This system has proven a lot credibility in prognosis and checking out due to its system of casting off contaminations even as leaving the wished samples for checking out.

Abnormal cytological specimens

Abnormal specimens from cervical smears are classified as: - High-grade squamous intraepithelial lesions (HGSIL); - Low-grade squamous intraepithelial lesions (LGSIL); - Abnormal squamous cells of unsure importance (ASC-US). The most common odd Pap smear locating is ASC-US, which debts for 5-10 in step with cent of all smears (Choma, 2003; Wilbur, 2003). On similarly research many girls with ASC-US don't have any enormous pathology or lesions. They may also happen a few signs and symptoms of the most cancers. In such instances the abnormality can be resulting from a circumstance that mimics cervical dysplasia, along with: - Cellular modifications because of tissue harm due to contamination, trauma or radiation; - Physiological modifications secondary to hormonal use and menopausal fame; - A extensive variety of artefacts attributable to education of the specimen (Choma and Wilbur, 2003). Seventy in line with cent [70%] of ASC-US and low-grade lesions solve spontaneously (Kubovchik, 2004). However, LGSIL or HGSIL warrant in addition research, usually through colposcopy and biopsy. In colposcopy the cervix is imaged and acetic acid implemented to spotlight ordinary epithelium. After software of acetic acid, atypical tissue will become deepwhite or brightened. Generally the extra intense the whitening, the extra intense the lesion. Where the rims of the lesion are in reality defined, vast ailment is greater probably.

Where the rims are fuzzy the adjustments are regularly induced with the aid of using viral change (Smith, 2000).

Usually a colposcopy completed after an extraordinary smear will screen a lesion from which a biopsy may be taken. Biopsies are graded the use of the cervical intraepithelial neoplasia (CIN) histological grading system, which quantifies diploma of mobile dysplasia rating from CIN I for slight dysplasia to III for superior dysplasia (Box 1). Most girls with LGSIL have CIN I sickness. This typically calls for no in addition remedy due to the fact ninety consistent with cent of CIN I abnormalities will now no longer development (Cooper et al, 2003) this is to mention it's miles self limiting. These girls are observed up with repeated smears and likely colposcopy (Cannistra and Niloff, 1996). CIN II or III ailment might be found in 5-10 consistent with cent of ladies with LGSIL. Women with HGSIL have a 70-seventy five in step with cent risk of a CIN II or III lesion and a 1-2 according to cent risk of invasive cervical most cancers (Wright et al, 2002). This shows that girls below this category [HGSIL] are in some way susceptible to having the lesion and must go to their hospital treatment employees if the any uncommon signs with their reproductive tract/organ.

Human papilloma virus

Almost all cervical cancers include strains of the human papilloma virus (HPV), which is likewise causative withinside the mobile modifications that result in ASC-US, LGSILs and HGSILs. It is idea to contaminate basal cells in the cervical epithelium gaining get entry to through minor trauma, or on the squamocolumnar junction (Cooper et al, 2003). There are sub-varieties of HPV: - Low threat - related to cutaneous contamination (together with warts) (HPV 6, 11, 40, 42, 43, 44); - High chance - related to infections of the genital tract (HPV 16, 18,

31, 33, 35, forty five); HPV 16, 18, 31 and forty five account for approximately eighty in step with cent of cervical cancers (Choma, 2003). About seventy five in keeping with cent of human beings of reproductive age were inflamed with HPV (Choma, 2003). Primary contamination happens primarily in younger adults, and a big percent of humans may be inflamed through the age of 30 (Helmerhorst and Meijer, 2002). The maximum vital hazard aspect for the purchase of HPV is range of sexual partners. HPV contamination is particularly asymptomatic and brief. Only 20 consistent with cent of human beings broaden premalignant lesions and most effective a small percent of those becomes cancerous. Ninety percent of infections remedy absolutely inside years with out identity of clinically huge lesions (Choma, 2003). It is uncertain if the virus is eliminated or simply suppressed to undctcctablc levels. Total abstinence from intercourse is the simplest manner to save you HPV contamination. Condoms provide a few protection, however now no longer if lesions stay uncovered. Also HPV can lie dormant for a while earlier than any signs and symptoms emerge as apparent. It is due to this affiliation with HPV that cervical most cancers is every now and then called a sexually transmitted ailment. However, whilst HPV is sexually transmitted, the mechanism wherein a malignancy develops isn't always. The occasion that transforms a brief contamination into mobile dysplasia or most cancers isn't always absolutely understood. Integration of HPV into the mobile genome is taken into consideration an crucial step withinside the procedure (Cooper et al, 2003). The immune reputation might be a huge issue. Thus a failure in immunosurveillance - possibly an expression of genetic defect - is simply as probably as life-style to be responsible. In current years it's been acknowledged that HPV checking out can be of importance withinside the control of low-grade lesions and ASC-US. A high quality HPV check with excessive-danger viral versions indicates extra competitive follow-up is warranted than if the virus is absent or is one of the low-grade strains. The US National Cancer Institute lately subsidized a big observe wherein an HPV check turned into discovered to be as powerful as repeat cervical smears for the control of ladies with ASC-US. This is now advocated via way of means of the American Society for Colposcopy and Cervical Pathology (Solomon et al, 2001), however has now no longer been recommended withinside the UK.

Managing precancerous lesions

CIN I lesions frequently clear up spontaneously, and are typically controlled via way of means of near observation, even as CIN II or III lesions require greater lively intervention. These variety from competitive techniques requiring clinic admission to much less competitive strategies that may be carried out as outpatient procedures. Treatment for CIN control has a ninety five percent of achievement price.

Excisional techniques

The conventional technique become to take a cone biopsy - the elimination of a cone-formed piece of tissue from the wall of the cervix. This 'bloodless knife' biopsy is much less not common nowadays however is on occasion used for CIN III lesions as it yields an amazing specimen for the pathologist to look at to decide that the surgical margins are clean. It normally necessitates sanatorium admission due to the comparatively massive quantity of cervical tissue removed. Where feasible cone biopsy has been changed through a much less complicated technique referred to as the loop electric powered excision of the transformation zone (LLETZ or LEEP), wherein the extraordinary tissue is excised the use of an tool composed of a cord heated through an electrical current. This may be carried out on an outpatient basis. The heated cord can motive a few harm to the margins of the biopsy specimen and isn't always utilised in instances wherein there may be situation approximately the histology on the excision margins.

Destructive techniques

The use of radical diathermy or cryotherapy is now limited. Cryotherapy is technically difficult. Laser remedy with a CO2 laser also can be technically tough. Immediate headaches of those remedies are ache and haemorrhage. Patients ought to keep away from sexual intercourse, tampons and douching till the incision is absolutely healed, which can also additionally take numerous weeks. A small variety of ladies revel in cervical stenosis. Post method girls require common smears or colposcopies, as decided through their gynaecologist (Smith, 2000).

Cervical cancers remedy

There are 4 levels of cervical most cancers, level 1 being the least invasive. Here the most cancers is restricted to the cervix while in degree four it extends to the bladder, rectum and remote sites (Box 1). Localised sickness is controlled through surgical operation. Widespread ailment can also additionally require radiotherapy, surgical treatment and chemotherapy. The 4-yr survival price from early cervical most cancers is ninety five according to cent, however drops to 0-39 consistent with cent with superior ailment (Rajaram, 1998).

Surgery

For localised ailment limited to the cervix, surgical procedure is the remedy of choice. Radiotherapy is similarly powerful however has a tendency to hold extra side-outcomes. Surgery entails a vaginal or belly hysterectomy. Vaginal hysterectomy is elimination of the uterus and cervix via the vagina. It is the much less stressful of the 2 however can be hard in people with different gynaecological issues or overweight sufferers. Abdominal hysterectomy includes surgical elimination of the uterus, higher a part of the vagina, ligaments and connective tissues that keep the uterus in region through an incision withinside the abdomen. Pelvic lymph nodes also are regularly resected, and an oophorectomy and salpingectomy can be required. Surgical tactics might also additionally result in some of lengthy-time period headaches, especially if radiotherapy is utilised as well. Bergmark et al (2002) determined sexual disorder to be a first-rate reason of distress, in addition to lymphoedema, dyspareunia and the pressing want to defecate. It is predicted that 10-15 in line with cent of cervical cancers are recognized in girls who're nevertheless inside their child-bearing years. The radical trachelectomy is a specialized surgery which permits upkeep of the frame of the uterus for younger ladies with early-level cervical most cancers. This is a extraordinarily new technique, and information is being gathered to set up its position (Plante and Roy, 2001). Radiotherapy

Radiation remedy has been used efficaciously to deal with carcinoma of the cervix because the early 1900s. Adjuvant radiotherapy is utilised if there's a threat of residual ailment post surgery.

Unfortunately, for the control of big cervical lesions the dose of radiation had to gain tumour manage exceeds the dose tolerated through the ordinary tissues of the pelvis. Tumour length is an vital predictor of outcome. As tumours growth in length they exceed their blood deliver and increase hypoxia and necrosis. This hypoxia outcomes in decreased efficacy of each radiotherapy and chemotherapy. Anaemia is notion to have a comparable impact and is consequently a bad prognostic element in cervical most cancers. Hyperthermia, neutron beam irradiation, interstitial brachytherapy and excessive-dose price intracavitary radiation had been investigated in reversing the consequences of hypoxia however have now no longer ended in predominant benefits (Rose, 2001). The maximum vast improvement in enhancing efficacy of radiotherapy is find of concurrent chemotherapy, which has been discovered to behave as a radiosensitiser. The remedies are concept to behave synergistically thru: - Simultaneous interest of drug and radiation in unique stages of the mobile cycle and towards exclusive tumour subpopulations; - Radiotherapy lowering tumour mobile repopulation; - Increased tumour cellular recruitment out of resting segment to responsive levels withinside the mobile cycle; - Inhibition of restore of sub-deadly radiation harm (Loizzi et al, 2003).

Chemotherapy

Disseminated disorder is often handled with the aid of using chemotherapy. Survival prices post recurrence are limited - approximately 30 in keeping with cent of sufferers die of recurrent sickness. Prognostic elements with a terrible effect on survival encompass: - Recurrence inside a formerly irradiated area; - Young age; - Poor overall performance reputation; - Short time to development from preliminary prognosis (Eralp et al, 2003). Cisplatin seems to be the maximum lively chemotherapy agent, with reaction quotes of approximately 20 according to cent. Some aggregate regimens that utilise a more wide variety of chemotherapy dealers had been located to yield better reaction costs (50-60 in line with cent), however this isn't always always pondered in accelerated survival. Furthermore, the employment of more than one sellers will increase the capability for toxicity, that is of precise importance amongst this population, whose analysis is poor (Eralp et al, 2003). Chemotherapy has additionally been investigated in adjuvant and neoadjuvant settings, however there's no compelling statistics to guide use of both routinely (Loizzi et al, 2003).

Increasing uptake of screening

Most ladies who expand cervical most cancers have by no means been often screened, both due to the fact they're residents of a rustic that lacks the infrastructure to offer such screening or due to the fact there are obstacles to their participation in a screening programme (O'Meara, 2002). Within evolved nations 30-eighty in line with cent of ladies identified with an extraordinary smear fail to go back for follow-up care (Rajaram, 1998). High-chance agencies consist of ladies belonging to minority ethnic companies, more youthful ladies, girls on decrease earning and people who're knowledgeable to under excessive-faculty level. These girls additionally revel in reduced survival quotes for cervical most cancers. For example, the mortality charge amongst African-Americans is two times that of white ladies (Choma, 2003). Lack of uptake of screening programmes through minority ethnic girls is a hassle. Chiu (2004) describes a assignment withinside the UK wherein girls and fitness experts have been concerned in studies to pick out and remedy the issues that stopped girls from participating. A key difficulty turned into issue in expertise and verbal exchange among the 2 businesses. Chiu observed a clean divergence among the perceptions of the smear-takers and people of the girls from minority ethnic organizations, which ended in bad studies on each sides. In the beyond there was an assumption that provision of data is the solution to uptake issues, however this paper diagnosed a urgent want to appearance extra. Close relationships frequently expand among nurses and their sufferers, and this locations them in a perfect state of affairs to teach girls approximately the cause and gain of cervical most cancers screening - especially amongst girls from excessive-hazard agencies. Current countrywide tips of screening tips are given in Box 2.

Conclusion

Cervical most cancers is declining in occurrence withinside the advanced world, and even though no randomised trials were done, it's miles idea that the screening programme is liable for this decline (Sedlacek, 2002). Treatment for superior most cancers stays tricky and has discouraging reaction fees. Management techniques have to depend upon early detection and screening thru programmes which are additionally suitable to girls who belong to minority ethnic corporations and who're at excessive chance. Nurses can play critical position in encouraging girls to take part withinside the NHS cervical screening programme